THE HEALING POWERS OF HONEY

EXPOSING THE HIDDEN MEDICINAL BENEFITS OF HONEY

BY Dr Benjamin James

Dr Benjamin James

Dr Benjamin James

Contents

Dr Benjamin James

HISTORY OF THE MEDICAL USES OF HONEY

Antibiotics have an essential role in reducing the global burden of infectious diseases. However, the efficacy deteriorates when resistant organisms arise and spread. Antimicrobial resistance poses a significant concern to public health, and resistance to all types of antibiotics, including the most used last-resort treatments, is on the rise worldwide.

As a result, alternative antibacterial approaches are desperately needed, prompting a reconsideration of the therapeutic use of ancient medicines such as plants and plant-based products like honey. Traditional medicine has been used to cure infection since the beginning of time, and honey made by Apis mellifera (A. mellifera) is one of the oldest traditional medicines still used to treat various human disorders.

Many studies have been conducted on honey's antibacterial action. It has been discovered that natural unheated honey exhibits some broad-spectrum antibacterial activity when tested against pathogenic bacteria, oral bacteria, and food spoilage bacteria.

Honey has been used for both nutritional and medicinal purposes in most ancient cultures. The belief that honey is a nutrient, a drug, and an ointment has persisted into modern times, and as a result, an alternative medicine branch known as apitherapy has emerged in recent years, offering treatments based on honey and other bee products for a variety of ailments, including bacterial infections. Currently, several kinds of honey are available with antibacterial activity levels that have been standardized. Around 60 types of bacteria, including aerobes and anaerobes, gram-positives and gram-negatives, have been reported to be inhibited by Leptospermum scoparium (L. scoparium) honey, the most well-known of the kinds of honey.

Tualang honey exhibits varied but broad-spectrum antibacterial activity against various wounds and gastrointestinal pathogens. The antibacterial activities of Leptospermum spp. honeys are light and heat stable, unlike glucose oxidase. Because of hydrogen peroxide, the effectiveness of antibacterial activities in natural honey from other sources can vary by up to 100-fold.

Honey is also hygroscopic, which means it can absorb moisture from the environment and dehydrate bacteria, and its high sugar content and low pH can inhibit the growth of microbes. Based upon the extensive searches in several biomedical science journals and web-based reports, we discussed the updated facts and phenomena related to the medicinal property of honeys with emphasis on their antibacterial activities in this review.

Dr Benjamin James

MEDICINAL PROPERTIES

Honey is an old therapy for treating infected wounds that have recently been "rediscovered" by the medical community, especially in cases where current therapeutic drugs fail. Honey's usage as medication and an ointment is mentioned in the first recorded reference to honey, dating back to 2100-2000 BC on a Sumerian tablet. When addressing different kinds of honey, Aristotle (384-322 BC) described pale honey as "useful as a balm for sore eyes and sores." Honey has been used to speed wound healing since ancient times, and the ability of honey to aid wound healing has been proved numerous times.

Honey is becoming more widely accepted as a treatment for ulcers, bedsores, and other skin infections caused by burns and wounds. Honey's healing properties are because to its antibacterial properties, ability to maintain a moist wound environment that promotes healing, and high viscosity, which helps to provide a protective barrier against infection. Honey has been reported to be particularly useful as a treatment for wounds, burns, skin ulcers, and inflammations. Honey's antibacterial characteristics speed up the creation of new tissue, allowing the lesion to heal faster. In vivo action has been demonstrated for medihoney and manuka honey, making them appropriate for treating ulcers, infected wounds, and burns.When used topically, honey clears wound infection quickly, allowing deep surgical wounds with infection to recover quickly. Honey can aid in healing infected wounds that do not respond to traditional treatment, such as antibiotics and antiseptics, such as wounds infected with methicillin-resistant bacteria. It can also be used successfully on skin grafts and infected skin graft donor sites.

Manuka, jelly bush, and pasture jars of honey have been shown to stimulate the secretion of TNF- by monocytes, the progenitors of macrophages. On the other hand, Glycosylated proteins can cause macrophages to secrete TNF, a cytokine that is known to trigger wound healing mechanisms. Honey's capacity to inhibit the release of "reactive intermediates" may also help to limit tissue damage caused by activated macrophages during wound healing.

Honey's immunomodulatory properties are thus relevant to wound healing. According to both traditional folklore and modern reports, honey has been used as a cure for gastric ulcers and gastritis for centuries. Honey has been shown to aid in the repair of the injured intestinal mucosa, stimulate tissue growth, and act as an anti-inflammatory agent. Raw honey includes a lot of antioxidant-like substances such as flavonoids and other polyphenols. When honey is given to wounds, clinical findings have shown that the symptoms of inflammation are alleviated. Exudate elimination in wounds dressed with honey aids in the management of inflamed wounds.

Manuka honey for example has been shown to have antibacterial activity against pathogenic bacteria, including Staphylococcus aureus (S. aureus) and Helicobacter pylori (H. pylori), making it a good functional diet for the digestive system.

HONEY AS AN ANTI BACTERIAL ACTIVITY

Honey is used as a traditional treatment for microbiological diseases since antiquity. Manuka (L. scoparium) honey has been shown to be effective against a variety of human infections, including Escherichia coli (E. coli), Enterobacter aerogenes, Salmonella typhimurium, and Staphylococcus aureus. Honey has been shown to be effective against methicillin-resistant S. aureus (MRSA), haemolytic streptococci, and vancomycin-resistant Enterococci (VRE) in laboratory studies. Due to increased antibacterial action, local production (thus availability), and improved selectivity against medically significant pathogens, the newly found kinds of honey may offer advantages over or commonalities with manuka honey. In their susceptibility to honey of equal antibacterial activity, coagulase-negative staphylococci are quite similar to S. aureus, and more susceptible than Pseudomonas aeruginosa (P. aeruginosa) and Enterococcus species[14].

The disc diffusion method is primarily a qualitative test for determining bacterial susceptibility to antimicrobial compounds; nevertheless, the minimum inhibitory concentration (MIC) represents the amount of antimicrobial agent required to inhibit bacteria. Honey has an antibacterial effect against germs that can cause life-threatening infections in humans like Septicemia, urinary infections, and wound infections caused by Proteus spp.

HONEY INHIBITION ZONE DIAMETER

The zone width of inhibition (ZDI) of different honey samples (5–20%) against E. coli O157: H7 (12 mm–24 mm) and S. typhimurium (0 mm–20 mm) has been determined. For S. aureus, P.

aeruginosa, and E. coli, the ZDIs of Nilgiris kinds of honey were reported to be (20–21) mm, (15-16) mm, and (13–14) mm, respectively. Agbagwa and Frank-Peterside compared the abilities of different honey samples, including Western Nigerian honey, Southern Nigerian honey, Eastern Nigerian honey, and Northern Nigerian honey, to inhibit the growth of S. aureus, P. aeruginosa, E. coli, and Proteus mirabilis (P. mirabilis) with ZDIs of (5.3–11.6) mm, (1.4–15.4) mm, (4.4–13. ZDI (6.94–37.94) mm was found in raw and processed honey extracts against gram-positive bacteria such as S. aureus, Bacillus subtilis, Bacillus cereus, and gram-negative bacteria such as E. coli, P. aeruginosa, and Salmonella enterica serovar Typhi. Based on the ZDI generated for clinical (C) MRSA and standard (S) MRSA, E. coli, and

P. aeruginosa isolates, antibacterial activity of ulmo and manuka honeys was determined.

HONEY INHIBITORY CONCENTRATION MINIMUM

For MRSA isolates, the MIC was found to be lower with ulmo (Eucryphia cordifolia) honey (3.1 percent – 6.3 percent v/v) than with manuka honey (12.5 percent v/v); for E. coli and Pseudomonas bacteria, the MICs were found to be equal (12.5 percent v/v). Tualang honey had MICs ranging from 8.75 percent to 25 percent, while manuka honey had MICs ranging from 8.75 percent to 20 percent against a variety of pathogenic gram-positive and gram-negative bacteria. Manuka, heather, khadikraft, and local honeys had MICs of 10% – 20%, 10% – 20%, 11%, and 10% – 20%, respectively, against clinical and environmental isolates of P.

aeruginosa. The MICs of A. mellifera honey (126.23 – 185.70 mg/mL) and Tetragonisca angustula honey (142.87 – 214.33) mg/mL against S. aureus were found to be (126.23 – 185.70) mg/mL and (142.87 – 214.33) mg/mL, respectively. For S. typhimurium and E. coli O157:H7, the Egyptian clover honey MIC was 100 mg/mL. For S. aureus, P. aeruginosa, and E. coli, the Nilgiri honey MICs were 25 percent, 35 percent, and 40 percent, respectively. S. aureus, B. subtilis, B. cereus, and gram-negative bacteria (E. coli, P. aeruginosa, and S. typhi) all had MIC values of (0.625–5.000) mg/mL for honey extracts.

The MICs of Tualang honey against wound and enteric bacteria ranged from 8.75 percent to 25 percent, compared to 8.75 percent to 20 percent for manuka honey. This kinds of honey were inhibitory against coagulase-negative bacteria at dilutions as low as 3.6 percent – 0.7 percent (v/v) for the pasture honey and 3.4 percent – 0.5 percent (v/v) for the manuka honey. Many publications have found the MICs of various types of honey for various harmful bacterial strains including oral bacterial strains and bacterial strains causing wound infections. This why varied honey kinds have different MICs for bacterial strains that cause wound infections.

TIME IN KILLING BACTERIA

The kill kinetics provide a more realistic picture of antibacterial activity than the MIC. The time-kill activity of autoclaved honey against E. coli, P. aeruginosa, and S. Typhi in order to determine the efficacy of a hitherto unstudied local honey gathered from a village in West Bengal, India was investigated. Antibiotic susceptible and resistant S. aureus, S. epidermidis, Enterococcus faecium, E. coli, P. aeruginosa, E. cloacae, and Klebsiella oxytoca isolates were killed by 10 percent –40 percent (v/v) honey within 24 hours. More research said to be needed to establish various local honeys based on kill kinetics and in vivo efficacy against MDR illnesses.

Honey's antibacterial properties are related to its high osmolarity, low pH(acidity), and amount of hydrogen peroxide (H_2O_2) and non-peroxide components, such as the existence of phytochemical components such as methylglyoxal (MGO). Honey's antimicrobial properties are mostly hydrogen peroxide, whose content is governed by relative quantities of glucose oxidase produced by bees and catalase derived from flower pollen. When diluted, most honey varieties produce H2O2 due to the activation of the enzyme glucose oxidase, which oxidizes glucose to gluconic acid and H2O2, resulting in antibacterial activity. However, heat or the presence of catalase can rapidly destroy the peroxide activity in honey in specific instances.

Aside from H2O2, which is created by the endogenous enzyme glucose oxidase in most typical jars of honey, numerous other non-peroxide components are responsible for honey's distinctive antibacterial activity. Honey can retain antibacterial activity even when catalase (glucose oxidase) is present, and this sort of honey is referred to as "non-peroxide honey". The presence of methyl syringate and methylglyoxal, which have been widely researched in manuka honey obtained from the manuka tree (L. scoparium), are known to contribute to the non-peroxide action. Unlike manuka honey, the activity of ulmo honey is largely due to H2O2 production. When tested in the presence of catalase, a 25 percent (v/v) solution of ulmo honey had no detectable antibacterial activity. In contrast, manuka honey retained its antibacterial activity at the same concentration (absence of H2O2). The sterilizing treatment of gamma-irradiation does not affect either sort of activity.

Honey is acidic with a pH from 3.2 to 4.5, which is low enough to suppress several bacterial pathogens; Figure 4 shows the pH values of various kinds of honey. Some common harmful bacteria require a minimum pH of 4.3 to grow: E. coli (4.3), Salmonella spp. Honey's antibacterial qualities are due to the osmotic impact of its high sugar content and low moisture content, as well as the acidic properties of gluconic acid and the antiseptic capabilities of H2O2. In a recent investigation of honey's antibacterial characteristics in vitro, researchers discovered that H2O2, MGO, and an antimicrobial peptide called bee defensin-1 are all implicated in honey's bactericidal activity. The antibacterial efficacy of different jars of honey might vary by more than 100 times, depending on their regional, seasonal, and botanical origins, as well as harvesting, processing, and storage circumstances. The antibacterial properties of honey rely on a number of parameters, the most important of which are H2O2, phenolic chemicals, wound pH, honey pH, and the osmotic pressure exerted by the honey. Honey's antibacterial activity is mostly due to hydrogen peroxide, and variable amounts of this molecule in different honeys result in diverse antimicrobial effects. Physical properties, geographical dispersion, and distinct floral sources have been suggested to play a role in honey's antibacterial activity. It has also been discovered that the antibacterial activity of different kinds of honey varies significantly depending on the plant source. Honey's antibacterial activity has been demonstrated to range from 3 percent to 50 percent and higher. Honey's bactericidal action is based on the amount of honey used and the type of bacteria. Honey's antibacterial action is affected by its concentration; the higher the concentration, the more effective honey is as an antibacterial agent.

Dr Benjamin James

In Conclusion

Manuka honey has been extensively studied, and its antibacterial properties are well-known around the world. Honey has never been found to have microbiological resistance, making it a promising topical antibacterial agent for treating antibiotic-resistant bacteria (e.g., MDR S. maltophilia) and persistent wound infections that do not respond to antibiotic therapy. As a result, honey has been utilized as a last-resort treatment. Honey's efficacy against germs, such as Tualang honey, suggests that it could be employed as an alternative medicinal agent in some medical diseases, such as wound infection.

Honey other than commercially available antibacterial honey (e.g., manuka honey) can exhibit equal antibacterial action against bacterial pathogens, according to Lusby et al. Tualang honey inhibits the growth of bacterial species that cause stomach illnesses, such as S. typhi, S. flexneri, and E. coli, at low concentrations. Tualang honey has been shown to be effective against E. coli, S. typhi, and S. pyogenes; therefore, when taken orally in its pure, unadulterated form, it may help speed up recovery from these infections. Honey works well as a glucose substitute in oral rehydration, and its antibacterial properties help to decrease the length of bacterial diarrhea.

Antimicrobial resistance developments in burn wound bacterial infections are currently posing a severe challenge. Thus, honey with antibacterial activities against antibiotic-resistant organisms such as MRSA and MDR P. aeruginosa, Acinetobacter spp., and members of the family

Enterobacteriaceae, which have been linked to burn wound infections and nosocomial infections, is highly anticipated.

Overall, due to differences in the in vitro bactericidal activity of diverse kinds of honey, the unpredictable antibacterial activity of non-standardized honey may stymie its adoption as an antimicrobial agent. Currently, several kinds of honey with regulated levels of antibacterial activity are offered, the most well-known of which are manuka (Leptospermum) and Tualang (Koompassia excelsa) honey. Because of its broad-spectrum bactericidal activity, medical-grade honey (Revamil, medihoney) should be evaluated for therapeutic use as a topical antibacterial prophylactic or treatment for topical infections caused by antibiotic-resistant as well as antibiotic-sensitive bacteria. Furthermore, at a concentration of 10% (v/v), mountain, manuka, capillano, and eco-honeys showed inhibitory activity against H. pylori isolates, suggesting that locally produced kinds of honey have high antibacterial activity equivalent to commercial jars of honey. As a result, other honey produced locally but not yet tested for an antibacterial activity must be investigated.

www.ingramcontent.com/pod-product-compliance
Lightning Source LLC
Chambersburg PA
CBHW072332270726
48658CB00016B/2374